Healthy and Delicious Smoothie Recipes for Breakfast

Health is wealth

Prince emmanuel

DEDICATION

This book is Dedicated to my Mentor Mrs Maureen
Emmanuel
And to my Dad Emmanuel

CONTENTS

1

INTRODUCTION

Welcome to "Healthy and Delicious Smoothie Recipes for Breakfast" – a delightful journey into the world of nutritious and scrumptious smoothies that will revitalize your mornings and set the tone for a vibrant day ahead. This eBook is a celebration of the art of blending wholesome ingredients into delectable concoctions, providing you with a treasure trove of mouthwatering recipes and essential tips to elevate your breakfast game.

Importance of a Healthy Breakfast:

Breakfast is often hailed as the most important meal of the day, and for good reason. It kickstarts your metabolism, replenishes your energy levels after a night of rest, and fuels your body for the day's activities. A well-balanced breakfast is crucial for maintaining concentration, promoting weight management, and supporting overall well-being.

However, in our busy lives, we may often neglect breakfast or settle for quick, unhealthy options. This eBook aims to change that by showcasing the wonders of smoothies as a wholesome and convenient breakfast choice. By incorporating nutrient-packed fruits, vegetables, and other nourishing ingredients into your morning routine, you can embark on a journey towards better health and vitality.

Benefits of Smoothies as Breakfast Options:

Smoothies offer a myriad of benefits that make them an ideal breakfast option for individuals of all ages and lifestyles:

- Nutrient-Rich: Packed with vitamins, minerals, and antioxidants, smoothies are a delicious way to infuse your body with essential nutrients from a variety of fruits and vegetables.

- Quick and Convenient: With busy mornings in mind, smoothies are a breeze to prepare and can be enjoyed on-the-go, ensuring you never skip breakfast again.
- Customizable: The versatility of smoothies allows for endless customization to suit your taste preferences and dietary requirements. Whether you crave something sweet, tangy, or savory, there's a smoothie for every palate.
- Satiating: Combining fruits, vegetables, and protein sources, smoothies are a satiating and satisfying breakfast that keeps hunger at bay until your next meal.
- Digestive Health: Blending ingredients breaks down fibers, making it easier for your body to absorb nutrients and support healthy digestion.

Overview of the Book's Content:

Within the pages of this eBook, you'll discover a diverse collection of delightful smoothie recipes that cater to a range of tastes and nutritional needs. From fruity delights that transport you to tropical paradises to nutrient-packed green elixirs that energize your body, our recipes are designed to excite your taste buds while nourishing your body.

The eBook is structured to guide you through various aspects of smoothie making:

- Chapter I: "Smoothie Basics" introduces you to the essential elements of crafting perfect smoothies, including understanding the nutritional components, selecting the right base, and choosing the perfect blender and other essential equipment.
- Chapter II: "Incorporating Superfoods" explores the wonders of nutrient-rich superfoods that enhance the health benefits of your smoothies, elevating them to new levels of nourishment.
- Chapter III: "Energizing Fruit-Based Smoothies" indulges your senses with a selection of vibrant fruit-based blends

that provide a burst of energy and a medley of flavors.

- And much more, as we journey through chapters dedicated to protein-packed smoothies, green and detoxifying elixirs, nut-free options, smoothie bowl creations, immune-boosting blends, kid-friendly favorites, and valuable tips for customizing your smoothies.

In this eBook, you'll find not only a collection of enticing recipes but also a wealth of knowledge and inspiration to make smoothies an integral part of your daily breakfast routine. Whether you're a seasoned smoothie enthusiast or just starting your culinary journey, these recipes are crafted to suit everyone's palate and dietary preferences.

Join us on this flavorful expedition, and embrace a healthier and more delightful breakfast experience with "Healthy and Delicious Smoothie Recipes for Breakfast." May these blends invigorate your mornings, nourish your body, and bring a smile to your face as you savor the goodness in every sip. Cheers to a breakfast of health, happiness, and endless smoothie possibilities!

Smoothie Basics

In this chapter, we delve into the essential elements of crafting perfect smoothies that will kickstart your day with a burst of nutrition and flavor. Understanding the smoothie basics is the key to creating delicious and wholesome blends that cater to your taste preferences and dietary needs. Let's explore the three fundamental aspects that form the foundation of our smoothie-making journey.

Understanding the Nutritional Components of Smoothies:

Smoothies are more than just a tasty beverage; they are a nutritional powerhouse that can provide a wide array of essential nutrients. To create a well-balanced smoothie, it's essential to understand the key nutritional components that go into the blend:

- Fruits: Incorporate a variety of fresh or frozen fruits to add natural sweetness, vitamins, minerals, and fiber. From bananas and berries to tropical delights like mangoes and pineapples, the possibilities are endless.

- Vegetables: Don't be afraid to sneak in nutrient-rich vegetables like spinach, kale, or carrots to enhance the nutritional profile of your smoothie. They add a subtle flavor while providing essential vitamins and antioxidants.

- Protein: Ensure your smoothie is satisfying and satiating by adding protein sources like Greek yogurt, nut butters, seeds, or protein powders. Protein promotes muscle repair, supports energy levels, and helps keep hunger at bay.

- Liquid Base: Choose a liquid base that complements the other ingredients, such as milk (dairy or plant-based), water, coconut water, or fruit juices. The liquid consistency can be adjusted to your preference.

- Healthy Fats: Add a dose of healthy fats from sources like avocados, nuts, or chia seeds, which not only contribute to a creamy texture but also offer numerous health benefits.

- Superfoods: For an extra boost of nutrition, experiment with superfoods like chia seeds, spirulina, maca powder, or acai berries. These powerhouse ingredients elevate your smoothie to a new level of nourishment.
Selecting the Right Base: Milk, Plant-Based Milk, Water, or Juice:

The liquid base of your smoothie plays a crucial role in determining the taste and texture of the final blend. The choice of liquid can also impact the nutritional content of your smoothie. Here are some popular options to consider:

- Milk: Dairy milk adds creaminess and a subtle richness to smoothies. It also provides calcium and protein. Opt for low-fat or non-dairy milk if you have dietary preferences or restrictions.

- Plant-Based Milk: For a vegan or lactose-free option, choose plant-based milks like almond milk, soy milk, coconut milk, or oat milk. These alternatives come in various flavors and add unique undertones to your smoothie.
- Water: For a light and refreshing smoothie, water is a great option. It allows the flavors of fruits and vegetables to shine through without overpowering the taste.
- Juice: Fruit juices like orange juice or apple juice can enhance the natural sweetness of your smoothie. However, be mindful of the added sugars in some commercial juices and opt for freshly squeezed or natural juices whenever possible.

Choosing the Perfect Blender and Other Essential Equipment:

The equipment you use can significantly impact the texture and consistency of your smoothie. Investing in the right blender and using other essential equipment will ensure smooth and luscious blends every time:

- Blender: Invest in a high-quality blender that can handle a variety of ingredients and blend them to a smooth and creamy texture. Look for blenders with sufficient power and variable speed settings to accommodate different ingredients.
- Cutting Board and Knife: A sturdy cutting board and sharp knife are essential for preparing fruits and vegetables for your smoothies. Properly washed and chopped ingredients ensure a smoother blending process.
- Measuring Cups: Accurate measurements are crucial to maintaining the right balance of ingredients and achieving the desired taste and texture. Use measuring cups or spoons to follow recipes precisely.
- Strainer or Nut Milk Bag: If you prefer a smoother texture and want to remove pulp or seeds, a fine mesh strainer or nut

milk bag can be handy for straining your smoothie.

- Mason Jars or Reusable Bottles: Prepare your smoothies in advance and store them in mason jars or reusable bottles for convenience on busy mornings. This way, you can grab a nutritious breakfast on the go.
- Ice Trays: To keep your smoothies chilled without diluting the flavor, freeze some of the liquid base in ice trays and use these ice cubes instead of regular ice.

By mastering the smoothie basics, you'll become a smoothie connoisseur, confidently crafting delicious and nutrient-packed blends that cater to your taste preferences and support your overall well-being. Armed with the right knowledge, ingredients, and equipment, you're ready to embark on a delightful and nourishing smoothie-making adventure!

3

Incorporating Superfoods

Welcome to the world of "Incorporating Superfoods" in your delightful smoothie creations. In this chapter of "Healthy and Delicious Smoothie Recipes for Breakfast," we embark on a journey to explore the wonders of superfoods, infusing your morning blends with an extra boost of nutrition and wellness. These nutrient-dense powerhouses are nature's gifts, providing a wide array of essential vitamins, minerals, antioxidants, and other health-promoting properties.

Exploring Nutrient-Rich Superfoods for Boosting Health:

Superfoods are renowned for their exceptional nutrient profiles and remarkable health benefits. In this section, we'll introduce you to a selection of nature's superheroes that will elevate your smoothies to nutritional heights:

- **Spirulina:** This vibrant blue-green algae is rich in protein, iron, B-vitamins, and antioxidants. Adding a teaspoon of spirulina powder to your smoothie not only enhances its nutritional content but also gives it a beautiful hue.
- **Maca Powder:** Derived from a root vegetable native to Peru, maca powder is known for its adaptogenic properties, supporting stress management and hormonal balance. It also provides essential minerals like calcium and potassium.
- **Chia Seeds:** These tiny seeds are packed with omega-3 fatty acids, fiber, and protein, promoting heart health and aiding digestion. When soaked, chia seeds create a gel-like consistency that adds a delightful texture to your smoothie.
- **Acai Berries:** Renowned for their deep purple hue, acai berries are rich in antioxidants, anthocyanins, and essential

fatty acids. They promote skin health and may help combat oxidative stress.

- **Hemp Seeds:** Hemp seeds are a complete protein source, offering all nine essential amino acids. They also provide a healthy balance of omega-3 and omega-6 fatty acids, benefiting cardiovascular health.
- **Cacao Nibs:** Derived from raw cacao beans, cacao nibs add a decadent chocolate flavor to your smoothies while offering antioxidants, iron, and magnesium.
- **Bee Pollen:** This natural treasure collected by bees is a source of vitamins, minerals, amino acids, and enzymes. It is believed to boost energy and support the immune system.

Adding Greens for Extra Nutrients and Energy:

Green smoothies are a fantastic way to incorporate nutrient-dense leafy greens into your breakfast routine. In this section, we'll explore various greens that effortlessly blend into your smoothies, enhancing both nutrition and taste:

- Spinach: Mild and versatile, spinach is an excellent source of iron, calcium, and vitamin K. Its mild flavor allows it to pair seamlessly with a variety of fruits.
- Kale: Rich in vitamins A, C, and K, kale adds a vibrant green color and earthy taste to your smoothie. It's a nutritional powerhouse that supports bone health and boosts the immune system.
- Swiss Chard: With its rainbow-colored stems, Swiss chard is not only visually appealing but also packed with vitamins and minerals, including magnesium, potassium, and vitamin C.
- Collard Greens: These robust leaves offer a dose of vitamin K, calcium, and folate. Blending them with fruits balances their slightly bitter taste.
- Romaine Lettuce: Light and refreshing, romaine lettuce provides vitamin A,

potassium, and folate. It's an excellent choice for those seeking a milder green flavor.

Incorporating Chia Seeds, Flaxseeds, and Hemp Seeds for Omega-3s:

Omega-3 fatty acids are essential for heart and brain health. In this section, we'll explore how chia seeds, flaxseeds, and hemp seeds add a dose of these healthy fats to your smoothies:

- **Chia Seeds:** These tiny seeds are a fantastic source of alpha-linolenic acid (ALA), a plant-based omega-3 fatty acid. They also provide fiber, protein, and essential minerals.
- **Flaxseeds:** Ground flaxseeds offer a rich source of ALA and lignans, which have antioxidant properties. When ground, flaxseeds release their nutrients for easier absorption.
- **Hemp Seeds:** Hemp seeds are unique for their ideal balance of omega-3 and omega-6 fatty acids. They support heart

health and may help reduce inflammation.

Incorporating superfoods into your smoothies not only boosts their nutritional value but also adds exciting flavors and textures to your morning ritual. These nutrient-rich additions empower you to seize the day with vitality and well-being. As you embark on your smoothie-making journey, feel free to experiment with various superfoods, greens, and omega-3 sources to create blends that resonate with your taste buds and nourish your body from the inside out.

Get ready to sip on a concoction of health and indulge in the magic of superfoods with every glorious sip of your smoothie. Cheers to a breakfast of health, happiness, and endless smoothie possibilities!

4

Energizing Fruit-Based Smoothies

In this chapter, we delve into a symphony of vibrant flavors and delightful combinations with our "Energizing Fruit-Based Smoothies." Bursting with the goodness of fresh and luscious fruits, these blends promise a refreshing start to your day, packed with vitamins, antioxidants, and natural sweetness. Embrace the power of nature's candy and let your taste buds dance to the melody of these nourishing elixirs.

Tropical Paradise: Mango, Pineapple, and Coconut Smoothie

Transport yourself to an exotic tropical paradise with this sunshine-filled smoothie. The combination of sweet mango, tangy pineapple, and creamy coconut milk creates a tropical symphony that will awaken your senses and leave you feeling rejuvenated.

Ingredients:

- 1 ripe mango, peeled and diced
- 1 cup fresh pineapple chunks
- 1 cup coconut milk
- 1 tablespoon honey or maple syrup (optional, for added sweetness)
- Ice cubes

Instructions:

Add the diced mango, pineapple chunks, and coconut milk to your blender.
If desired, add honey or maple syrup for a touch of sweetness.
Blend until smooth and creamy.
Add ice cubes and blend again until the smoothie is chilled.
Pour into a glass and garnish with a slice of fresh pineapple or a sprinkle of shredded coconut.

Berry Burst: Mixed Berry and Spinach Smoothie

Indulge in a burst of berry goodness with this vibrant and nutrient-rich smoothie. Packed with antioxidants, vitamins, and a handful of fresh spinach for an added health boost, this blend is a delectable way to start your day on a high note.

Ingredients:

- 1 cup mixed berries (strawberries, blueberries, raspberries, etc.)
- 1 ripe banana
- 1 cup fresh spinach leaves
- 1 cup almond milk (or any milk of your choice)
- 1 tablespoon chia seeds (optional, for extra nutrition)
- Ice cubes

Instructions:

Combine the mixed berries, ripe banana, fresh spinach, and almond milk in your blender.

If desired, add chia seeds for an extra nutritional punch.

Blend until the smoothie reaches a velvety consistency.

Add ice cubes and blend again until the smoothie is chilled.

Pour into a glass and garnish with a sprinkle of chia seeds or a few fresh berries.

Citrus Zest: Orange, Banana, and Turmeric Smoothie

Infuse your mornings with a burst of citrusy freshness and a touch of golden goodness with this zesty smoothie. The combination of sweet oranges, creamy banana, and anti-inflammatory turmeric makes for a rejuvenating and immune-boosting blend.

Ingredients:

- 2 ripe oranges, peeled and segmented

- 1 ripe banana
- 1/2 teaspoon ground turmeric
- 1 cup Greek yogurt (or any yogurt of your choice)
- 1 tablespoon honey (optional, for added sweetness)
- Ice cubes

Instructions:

Add the peeled and segmented oranges, ripe banana, ground turmeric, and Greek yogurt to your blender.

If desired, add honey for a touch of sweetness.

Blend until the smoothie reaches a velvety consistency.

Add ice cubes and blend again until the smoothie is chilled.

Pour into a glass and garnish with a slice of orange or a sprinkle of turmeric.

Embrace the invigorating taste of these fruit-based smoothies as they transport you to a world of delightful flavors and abundant nourishment. With each sip, you'll experience a burst of energy that will keep you fueled throughout the day. Feel free to customize these recipes with your favorite fruits or add a handful of spinach or kale for an extra nutritional boost. Energize your mornings and embrace the power of nature's bounty with our "Energizing Fruit-Based Smoothies."

I have condensed the chapter due to the character limit. If you need further elaboration or additional recipes, feel free to ask.

5

Protein-Packed Smoothies

In this chapter, we venture into the realm of "Protein-Packed Smoothies" – a collection of delectable blends that infuse your morning routine with a substantial dose of protein. These creations are designed to energize your body, support muscle repair, and keep you feeling satisfied until your next meal. Embrace the power of plant-based and dairy protein sources as we unveil these delicious and nutritious elixirs.

Creamy Peanut Butter Banana Smoothie

Indulge in the timeless combination of creamy peanut butter and ripe banana with this protein-packed delight. Packed with plant-based protein and healthy fats, this smoothie is a satisfying breakfast option that will leave you feeling nourished and ready to conquer the day.

Ingredients:

- 1 ripe banana
- 2 tablespoons natural peanut butter
- 1 cup milk of your choice (dairy or plant-based)
- 1 tablespoon honey or maple syrup (optional, for added sweetness)
- 1 tablespoon chia seeds (optional, for extra nutrition)
- Ice cubes

Instructions:

Peel the ripe banana and add it to your blender.

Add the natural peanut butter and milk of your choice.

If desired, add honey or maple syrup for a touch of sweetness.

For an extra nutritional boost, add chia seeds.

Blend until the smoothie reaches a velvety consistency.

Add ice cubes and blend again until the smoothie is chilled.

Pour into a glass and garnish with a drizzle of peanut butter or a sprinkle of chia seeds.
Almond Joy: Almond Milk, Cocoa, and Almond Butter Smoothie

Transport yourself to paradise with this protein-packed tribute to the classic Almond Joy flavor. The combination of almond milk, cocoa, and almond butter creates a rich and indulgent smoothie that satisfies your taste buds while nourishing your body with plant-based protein and essential nutrients.

Ingredients:

- 1 cup unsweetened almond milk
- 2 tablespoons almond butter
- 1 tablespoon unsweetened cocoa powder
- 1 ripe banana
- 1 tablespoon honey or maple syrup (optional, for added sweetness)
- Ice cubes

Instructions:

Pour the unsweetened almond milk into your blender.

Add almond butter and unsweetened cocoa powder.

Peel the ripe banana and add it to the blender.

If desired, add honey or maple syrup for a touch of sweetness.

Blend until the smoothie reaches a velvety consistency.

Add ice cubes and blend again until the smoothie is chilled.

Pour into a glass and garnish with a sprinkle of cocoa powder or a few slivered almonds.

Vanilla Berry Protein Smoothie with Greek Yogurt

Indulge in a burst of berry goodness and the creaminess of Greek yogurt with this protein-packed smoothie. The combination of sweet berries and vanilla-infused Greek yogurt creates a delightful and satisfying blend that fuels your body with high-quality protein.

Ingredients:

- 1 cup mixed berries (strawberries, blueberries, raspberries, etc.)
- 1 cup plain Greek yogurt
- 1 tablespoon honey or maple syrup (optional, for added sweetness)
- 1 teaspoon vanilla extract
- Ice cubes

Instructions:

Combine the mixed berries and plain Greek yogurt in your blender.

If desired, add honey or maple syrup for a touch of sweetness.

Add vanilla extract for a delightful flavor.

Blend until the smoothie reaches a velvety consistency.

Add ice cubes and blend again until the smoothie is chilled.

Pour into a glass and garnish with a few fresh berries or a drizzle of honey.

Embrace the protein-packed power of these smoothies and revel in the delightful flavors they bring to your breakfast table. These recipes are not only delicious but also nourishing, ensuring you start your day on the right foot and stay energized throughout your morning activities. Customize these blends with your favorite protein sources and explore different flavor combinations to suit your palate and dietary needs. With our "Protein-Packed Smoothies," you'll be armed with a satisfying and wholesome breakfast option that supports your active lifestyle and keeps your taste buds dancing.

I have condensed the chapter due to the character limit. If you need further elaboration or additional recipes, feel free to ask.

6

Green and Detoxifying Smoothies

In this chapter, we embrace the goodness of green and detoxifying ingredients, crafting a collection of "Green and Detoxifying Smoothies" that rejuvenate and revitalize your body. These nutrient-rich blends are packed with leafy greens, vibrant vegetables, and cleansing herbs to promote inner balance, enhance digestion, and support your body's natural detoxification process. Let these refreshing and invigorating smoothies be your secret weapon for a nourishing breakfast that sets the tone for a healthy day ahead.

Kale, Cucumber, and Green Apple Detox Smoothie

Start your day with a burst of green goodness with this revitalizing detox smoothie. Kale, cucumber, and green apple come together to create a refreshing blend that supports your body's detoxification processes and boosts your energy levels.

Ingredients:

- 1 cup chopped kale leaves (stems removed)
- 1 small cucumber, peeled and chopped
- 1 green apple, cored and chopped
- 1 tablespoon fresh lemon juice
- 1 tablespoon fresh ginger, grated
- 1 cup coconut water (or water)
- Ice cubes

Instructions:

Add the chopped kale leaves, cucumber, green apple, fresh lemon juice, and grated ginger to your blender.
Pour in the coconut water (or water) to help blend the ingredients smoothly.
Blend until the smoothie reaches a velvety consistency.

Add ice cubes and blend again until the smoothie is chilled.

Pour into a glass and garnish with a slice of cucumber or a sprinkle of chia seeds.

Spinach, Avocado, and Kiwi Green Energy Smoothie

Energize your morning with this vibrant green energy smoothie. The combination of spinach, creamy avocado, and zesty kiwi provides a powerful dose of vitamins, minerals, and healthy fats, giving you the fuel you need to conquer the day ahead.

Ingredients:

- 1 cup fresh spinach leaves
- 1 ripe avocado, peeled and pitted
- 2 kiwis, peeled and chopped
- 1 tablespoon honey or maple syrup (optional, for added sweetness)
- 1 cup almond milk (or any milk of your choice)
- Ice cubes

Instructions:

Combine the fresh spinach leaves, ripe avocado, and chopped kiwis in your blender.

If desired, add honey or maple syrup for a touch of sweetness.

Pour in the almond milk (or any milk of your choice) to help blend the ingredients smoothly.

Blend until the smoothie reaches a velvety consistency.

Add ice cubes and blend again until the smoothie is chilled.

Pour into a glass and garnish with a slice of kiwi or a sprinkle of hemp seeds.

Detox Green Smoothie with Lemon and Ginger

Refresh and cleanse your body with this zingy detox green smoothie. The combination of nutrient-packed greens, zesty lemon, and invigorating ginger creates a rejuvenating blend that helps flush out toxins and boost your immune system.

Ingredients:

- 1 cup baby spinach
- 1 cup kale leaves (stems removed)
- 1 cucumber, peeled and chopped
- 1 green apple, cored and chopped
- Juice of 1 lemon
- 1 tablespoon fresh ginger, grated
- 1 cup coconut water (or water)
- Ice cubes

Instructions:

Add the baby spinach, kale leaves, chopped cucumber, chopped green apple, lemon juice, and grated ginger to your blender.

Pour in the coconut water (or water) to help blend the ingredients smoothly.

Blend until the smoothie reaches a velvety consistency.

Add ice cubes and blend again until the smoothie is chilled.

Pour into a glass and garnish with a lemon slice or a few fresh mint leaves.

Embrace the power of greens and detoxifying ingredients with our "Green and Detoxifying Smoothies." These revitalizing blends are not only delicious but also nourishing, giving your body a gentle detox while providing essential vitamins and minerals. Customize these recipes with your favorite greens or herbs to create your unique combination of cleansing goodness. With these invigorating smoothies in your breakfast repertoire, you'll be ready to embark on a day filled with vibrancy and wellness.

I have condensed the chapter due to the character limit. If you need further elaboration or additional recipes, feel free to ask.

7

Nut-Free Options

In this chapter, we cater to those with nut allergies or sensitivities by presenting a collection of "Nut-Free Options" – smoothies that are equally delicious and nutritious without any nuts. These delightful blends rely on alternative ingredients to deliver the same creamy texture and mouthwatering flavors without compromising on taste or health benefits. Whether you have nut allergies or simply prefer nut-free variations, these smoothies are sure to satisfy your palate and energize your morning.

Creamy Coconut Milk and Banana Smoothie

Indulge in the tropical goodness of coconut with this creamy and satisfying smoothie. Coconut milk offers a luscious, nut-free alternative to traditional nut-based milks, and when combined with sweet bananas, it creates a rich and velvety blend that's perfect for a breakfast treat.

Ingredients:

- 2 ripe bananas
- 1 cup coconut milk
- 1 tablespoon honey or maple syrup (optional, for added sweetness)
- 1 teaspoon vanilla extract
- Ice cubes

Instructions:

Peel the ripe bananas and add them to your blender.
Pour in the coconut milk, vanilla extract, and optional honey or maple syrup.
Blend until the smoothie reaches a velvety consistency.
Add ice cubes and blend again until the smoothie is chilled.
Pour into a glass and garnish with a sprinkle of shredded coconut or a banana slice.

Blueberry Oat Smoothie with Soy Milk

This nutrient-packed smoothie combines the goodness of blueberries and fiber-rich oats with the creaminess of soy milk. Soy milk provides a nut-free and plant-based alternative that contributes to a smooth and satisfying texture.

Ingredients:

- 1 cup blueberries (fresh or frozen)
- 1/2 cup rolled oats
- 1 cup soy milk
- 1 tablespoon honey or maple syrup (optional, for added sweetness)
- Ice cubes

Instructions:

Add the blueberries, rolled oats, and soy milk to your blender.
If desired, add honey or maple syrup for a touch of sweetness.
Blend until the smoothie reaches a velvety consistency.

Add ice cubes and blend again until the smoothie is chilled.

Pour into a glass and garnish with a few fresh blueberries or a sprinkle of oats.

Raspberry Vanilla Smoothie with Rice Milk

Delight in the sweet and tart flavors of raspberries with this refreshing smoothie. Rice milk offers a nut-free and dairy-free base that pairs beautifully with the burst of raspberry goodness.

Ingredients:

- 1 cup raspberries (fresh or frozen)
- 1 cup rice milk
- 1 tablespoon honey or maple syrup (optional, for added sweetness)
- 1 teaspoon vanilla extract
- Ice cubes

Instructions:

Add the raspberries, rice milk, vanilla extract, and optional honey or maple syrup to your blender.
Blend until the smoothie reaches a velvety consistency.
Add ice cubes and blend again until the smoothie is chilled.
Pour into a glass and garnish with a few fresh raspberries or a drizzle of honey.

Indulge in the nut-free goodness of these smoothies, embracing alternative ingredients that create the same creamy and delicious results. Whether you have nut allergies, dietary preferences, or simply want to try new flavors, these "Nut-Free Options" provide a delightful way to start your day on a wholesome note. Customize these recipes with your favorite fruits and milk alternatives, and let your creativity shine as you explore the world of nut-free smoothie creations.

8

Smoothie Bowl Creations

In this chapter, we explore the delightful world of "Smoothie Bowl Creations" – a fusion of smoothies and bowls that combine the refreshing taste of a smoothie with the delightful texture of a bowl. These creations not only fuel your body with essential nutrients but also engage your senses with their vibrant colors and tantalizing toppings. Elevate your breakfast experience with these artful and nutritious smoothie bowls.

Acai Berry Bowl with Granola and Fresh Fruits

Indulge in the popular acai berry, a superfood that's rich in antioxidants and bursting with flavor. This vibrant bowl combines acai with a medley of fresh fruits and crunchy granola, offering a delightful contrast of textures and a burst of colors.

Ingredients:

- 2 packs frozen acai puree (unsweetened)
- 1 ripe banana
- 1/2 cup mixed berries (strawberries, blueberries, raspberries, etc.)
- 1/4 cup granola
- Fresh fruit slices (kiwi, berries, banana, etc.)
- Coconut flakes
- Chia seeds

Instructions:

In a blender, blend the frozen acai puree, ripe banana, and mixed berries until smooth and creamy.
Pour the smoothie into a bowl.
Top the smoothie with granola, fresh fruit slices, coconut flakes, and a sprinkle of chia seeds for added crunch and nutrition.
Enjoy the delightful taste and texture of this Acai Berry Bowl.

Green Goddess Smoothie Bowl with Nuts and Seeds

Elevate your breakfast with this Green Goddess Smoothie Bowl that's packed with greens, healthy fats, and protein-rich nuts and seeds. This invigorating bowl will leave you feeling energized and ready to tackle the day.

Ingredients:

- 1 cup baby spinach
- 1 ripe avocado
- 1/2 cup cucumber, chopped
- 1/2 cup pineapple chunks
- 1/4 cup almond milk
- 1 tablespoon chia seeds
- 1 tablespoon hemp seeds
- 1 tablespoon flaxseeds
- Sliced almonds
- Fresh mint leaves

Instructions:

In a blender, blend the baby spinach, ripe avocado, chopped cucumber, pineapple chunks, and almond milk until smooth and creamy.

Pour the smoothie into a bowl.

Top the smoothie with chia seeds, hemp seeds, flaxseeds, sliced almonds, and fresh mint leaves for an extra boost of nutrients and delightful crunch.

Savor the refreshing taste and satisfying texture of this Green Goddess Smoothie Bowl.

Dragon Fruit Smoothie Bowl with Coconut Flakes and Chia Seeds

Immerse yourself in the stunning beauty and unique taste of dragon fruit with this visually appealing and delicious smoothie bowl. The vibrant pink hue and delightful toppings make this bowl a feast for both the eyes and the taste buds.

Ingredients:

- 1 cup dragon fruit (fresh or frozen), cubed
- 1 ripe banana
- 1/2 cup coconut water

- 1 tablespoon honey or maple syrup (optional, for added sweetness)
- Fresh fruit slices (kiwi, berries, etc.)
- Coconut flakes
- Chia seeds

Instructions:

In a blender, blend the dragon fruit, ripe banana, and coconut water until smooth and creamy.
Pour the smoothie into a bowl.
Top the smoothie with fresh fruit slices, coconut flakes, and a sprinkle of chia seeds for a delightful burst of flavors and textures.
Relish the visual and culinary treat of this Dragon Fruit Smoothie Bowl.

Immerse yourself in the artistry and flavors of these Smoothie Bowl Creations. These bowls not only offer a delicious and nutritious breakfast but also provide an opportunity for creative expression as you decorate and arrange the toppings to your liking. Experiment with different fruits, nuts, seeds, and superfood powders to craft your perfect smoothie bowl. Let these vibrant and nourishing bowls transform your breakfast routine into a delightful and wholesome experience.

9

Energizing and Immune-Boosting Smoothies

IN THIS CHAPTER, WE UNVEIL A COLLECTION OF "ENERGIZING AND IMMUNE-BOOSTING SMOOTHIES" — BLENDS THAT INFUSE YOUR MORNINGS WITH A BURST OF VITALITY AND STRENGTHEN YOUR IMMUNE SYSTEM TO TACKLE THE CHALLENGES OF THE DAY. THESE SMOOTHIES ARE CRAFTED WITH NUTRIENT-DENSE INGREDIENTS AND POWERFUL SUPERFOODS THAT SUPPORT YOUR OVERALL WELL-BEING WHILE TANTALIZING YOUR TASTE BUDS. SUPERCHARGE YOUR BREAKFAST WITH THESE INVIGORATING AND IMMUNE-BOOSTING ELIXIRS.

COFFEE LOVER'S WAKE-UP SMOOTHIE

FOR THE COFFEE AFICIONADOS SEEKING A NUTRITIOUS ALTERNATIVE, THIS SMOOTHIE PROVIDES THE PERFECT BALANCE OF ENERGY AND HEALTH BENEFITS. PACKED WITH ANTIOXIDANTS AND NATURAL CAFFEINE, THIS COFFEE LOVER'S WAKE-UP SMOOTHIE IS SURE TO KICKSTART YOUR DAY WITH A JOLT OF INVIGORATION.

INGREDIENTS:

- 1 RIPE BANANA
- 1 CUP BREWED COFFEE (CHILLED)
- 1/2 CUP PLAIN GREEK YOGURT
- 1 TABLESPOON ALMOND BUTTER
- 1 TABLESPOON HONEY OR MAPLE SYRUP (OPTIONAL, FOR ADDED SWEETNESS)
- ICE CUBES

INSTRUCTIONS:

PEEL THE RIPE BANANA AND ADD IT TO YOUR BLENDER.

POUR IN THE CHILLED BREWED COFFEE, PLAIN GREEK YOGURT, ALMOND BUTTER, AND OPTIONAL HONEY OR MAPLE SYRUP.

Blend until the smoothie reaches a velvety consistency.

Add ice cubes and blend again until the smoothie is chilled.

Pour into a glass and garnish with a sprinkle of cocoa powder or a few coffee beans.

Immunity Booster: Orange, Carrot, and Turmeric Smoothie

Boost your immune system with this vibrant and nutritious smoothie. Oranges and carrots are rich in vitamin C, while turmeric adds anti-inflammatory properties to the mix, making this Immunity Booster smoothie a powerhouse for your overall health.

Ingredients:

- 2 large oranges, peeled and deseeded
- 1 large carrot, peeled and chopped
- 1-inch piece of fresh turmeric, peeled and grated (or 1 teaspoon ground turmeric)
- 1/2 cup coconut water (or water)
- 1 tablespoon honey or maple syrup (optional, for added sweetness)
- Ice cubes

INSTRUCTIONS:

ADD THE PEELED AND DESEEDED ORANGES, CHOPPED CARROT, GRATED TURMERIC (OR GROUND TURMERIC), AND COCONUT WATER TO YOUR BLENDER.

IF DESIRED, ADD HONEY OR MAPLE SYRUP FOR A TOUCH OF SWEETNESS.

BLEND UNTIL THE SMOOTHIE REACHES A VELVETY CONSISTENCY.

ADD ICE CUBES AND BLEND AGAIN UNTIL THE SMOOTHIE IS CHILLED.

POUR INTO A GLASS AND GARNISH WITH A SLICE OF ORANGE OR A SPRINKLE OF TURMERIC.

POMEGRANATE POWER SMOOTHIE WITH SPINACH AND GINGER

EXPERIENCE THE POWER OF POMEGRANATE, SPINACH, AND GINGER IN THIS ANTIOXIDANT-RICH SMOOTHIE. POMEGRANATES ARE KNOWN FOR THEIR POTENT HEALTH BENEFITS, AND WHEN COMBINED WITH NUTRIENT-DENSE SPINACH AND ZESTY GINGER, THIS SMOOTHIE BECOMES A TASTY AND IMMUNE-BOOSTING TREAT.

INGREDIENTS:

- 1 CUP POMEGRANATE ARILS (SEEDS)
- 1 CUP BABY SPINACH
- 1-INCH PIECE OF FRESH GINGER, PEELED AND GRATED
- 1 TABLESPOON CHIA SEEDS
- 1 CUP ALMOND MILK (OR ANY MILK OF YOUR CHOICE)
- ICE CUBES

INSTRUCTIONS:

COMBINE THE POMEGRANATE ARILS, BABY SPINACH, GRATED GINGER, CHIA SEEDS, AND ALMOND MILK IN YOUR BLENDER.

BLEND UNTIL THE SMOOTHIE REACHES A VELVETY CONSISTENCY.

ADD ICE CUBES AND BLEND AGAIN UNTIL THE SMOOTHIE IS CHILLED.

POUR INTO A GLASS AND GARNISH WITH A FEW POMEGRANATE ARILS OR A SPRINKLE OF CHIA SEEDS.

EMBRACE THE ENERGY AND IMMUNITY-BOOSTING BENEFITS OF THESE SMOOTHIES, EACH CAREFULLY CURATED TO NOURISH AND STRENGTHEN YOUR BODY. FROM THE COFFEE LOVER'S WAKE-UP SMOOTHIE TO THE VIBRANT IMMUNITY BOOSTER AND THE POMEGRANATE POWER SMOOTHIE, THESE RECIPES SHOWCASE THE DELICIOUS HARMONY OF

INGREDIENTS THAT INVIGORATE AND PROTECT. INCORPORATE THESE ENERGIZING AND IMMUNE-BOOSTING ELIXIRS INTO YOUR BREAKFAST ROUTINE AND WITNESS THE POSITIVE IMPACT THEY HAVE ON YOUR OVERALL WELL-BEING.

10

Kid-Friendly Smoothies

In this chapter, we embark on a journey to create "Kid-Friendly Smoothies" – delightful blends that not only appeal to young taste buds but also provide essential nutrients to support their growth and development. Packed with colorful fruits, hidden veggies, and natural sweetness, these smoothies are sure to become your child's favorite breakfast treat.

Sneaky Veggie Blueberry Smoothie

For parents who want to sneak in some veggies without their kids noticing, this smoothie is a winner. Blending nutrient-rich spinach with sweet blueberries, this Sneaky Veggie Blueberry Smoothie offers the best of both worlds – taste and nutrition.

Ingredients:

- 1 cup fresh spinach leaves
- 1 cup blueberries (fresh or frozen)
- 1 ripe banana
- 1/2 cup plain Greek yogurt
- 1 tablespoon honey or maple syrup (optional, for added sweetness)
- 1/2 cup milk (any variety)

Instructions:

In a blender, blend the fresh spinach leaves, blueberries, ripe banana, and plain Greek yogurt until smooth and creamy.
If desired, add honey or maple syrup for a touch of sweetness.

Pour in the milk of your choice to help blend the ingredients smoothly.
Blend again until the smoothie reaches a velvety consistency.
Pour into a kid-friendly cup and garnish with a blueberry or a fun straw.
Banana Split Smoothie: Chocolate, Banana, and Strawberry

Capture the essence of a classic banana split in a healthy smoothie form. This Banana Split Smoothie combines the irresistible flavors of chocolate, banana, and strawberry, making it a delightful treat for kids of all ages.

Ingredients:

- 2 ripe bananas
- 1 cup strawberries (fresh or frozen)
- 1 tablespoon cocoa powder
- 1 tablespoon almond butter (or peanut butter)
- 1 cup milk (any variety)
- Ice cubes

Instructions:

Peel the ripe bananas and add them to your blender.

Add the strawberries, cocoa powder, almond butter, and milk to the blender as well.

Blend until the smoothie reaches a velvety consistency.

Add ice cubes and blend again until the smoothie is chilled.

Pour into a kid-friendly cup and garnish with a strawberry slice or a drizzle of chocolate sauce.

PB&J Smoothie with Mixed Berries and Peanut Butter

Combining the classic flavors of peanut butter and jelly, this smoothie brings nostalgia and wholesomeness to the breakfast table. Packed with mixed berries and protein-rich peanut butter, the PB&J Smoothie is a nutritious twist on a beloved childhood favorite.

Ingredients:

- 1 cup mixed berries (strawberries, blueberries, raspberries)
- 1 ripe banana
- 1 tablespoon peanut butter
- 1 tablespoon honey or maple syrup (optional, for added sweetness)
- 1 cup milk (any variety)
- Ice cubes

Instructions:

Combine the mixed berries, ripe banana, peanut butter, and milk in your blender.
If desired, add honey or maple syrup for a touch of sweetness.
Blend until the smoothie reaches a velvety consistency.
Add ice cubes and blend again until the smoothie is chilled.
Pour into a kid-friendly cup and garnish with a berry or a peanut butter drizzle.

Introduce your little ones to the joy of wholesome breakfasts with these Kid-Friendly Smoothies. The vibrant colors, delicious flavors, and nutrient-rich ingredients will make breakfast an enjoyable experience for both kids and parents. Encourage your children to get creative by selecting their favorite fruits and experimenting with different combinations. With these delightful smoothies in their morning routine, kids will start their day with a smile and the energy they need to take on any adventure that comes their way.

11

Tips for Customizing Your Smoothies

In this chapter, we delve into the art of customization, offering valuable insights and "Tips for Customizing Your Smoothies." Embrace your creativity and preferences to craft the perfect smoothie tailored to your taste and nutritional needs. With a vast array of ingredients and combinations, these tips will empower you to create smoothies that suit your unique palate and promote a healthier lifestyle.

Adjusting Sweetness Levels and Flavor Profiles

One of the beauties of making smoothies at home is the flexibility to control the sweetness and flavor according to your liking. Here are some tips to achieve the perfect balance:

- Natural Sweeteners: Instead of refined sugars, opt for natural sweeteners like honey, maple syrup, agave nectar, or dates. These add a touch of sweetness without compromising on health.

- Fruits: The ripeness and sweetness of fruits can vary. Experiment with different fruits and their quantities to find the desired level of sweetness.
- Tartness: If your smoothie turns out too sweet, add a squeeze of lemon or lime juice to balance the flavors.
- Spices: Enhance the taste with a pinch of cinnamon, nutmeg, or vanilla extract for a warm and comforting flavor profile. Incorporating Protein Powders and Supplements

Smoothies provide an excellent canvas to incorporate protein powders and various nutritional supplements. Whether you aim to boost muscle recovery or increase your daily protein intake, these tips will guide you:

- Protein Powders: Explore different protein sources like whey, pea, hemp, or soy protein powders. They enrich your smoothie with essential amino acids and can cater to specific dietary preferences.

- Greek Yogurt: For a natural protein boost, Greek yogurt is an excellent addition. It also lends a creamy texture to the smoothie.
- Nut Butters: Incorporate almond butter, peanut butter, or other nut butters for a protein-rich and velvety smoothie.
- Seeds: Chia seeds, hemp seeds, and flaxseeds are not only great sources of protein but also provide a boost of fiber and healthy fats.
- Superfood Supplements: Enhance the nutritional value of your smoothie by adding superfood powders like spirulina, maca, or matcha.

Experimenting with Texture and Consistency

Smoothies offer endless possibilities for achieving the desired texture and consistency. Consider the following tips to customize your smoothie's texture:

- Ice: Add ice cubes to your blender to create a chilled and refreshing smoothie.

- Frozen Fruits: Replace fresh fruits with frozen alternatives to achieve a thicker and creamier texture.
- Thickeners: Avocado, frozen banana, cooked sweet potato, or oats act as natural thickeners and impart a luscious texture.
- Liquid Ratios: Adjust the amount of liquid (water, milk, juice, or plant-based milk) to achieve your preferred thickness.
- Blend Times: Blend for a shorter time for a chunkier smoothie or blend longer for a silky-smooth consistency.
- Garnishes: Top your smoothie with granola, shredded coconut, or crushed nuts for an added crunch and visual appeal.

Customize Your Smoothie Journey

Embrace the joy of customization and make each smoothie a reflection of your taste and nutritional goals. With these "Tips for Customizing Your Smoothies," you hold the key to an array of flavors and textures that will excite your taste buds and elevate your breakfast experience. Get creative, experiment with various ingredients, and let your smoothie journey be a delightful expression of your unique preferences and well-being.

12

Conclusion

Congratulations! You've embarked on a journey of flavor, nourishment, and creativity with "Healthy and Delicious Smoothie Recipes for Breakfast." This eBook has been crafted to bring you a delightful breakfast experience, replete with nutrient-rich ingredients and invigorating flavors. As we draw this culinary adventure to a close, let's reflect on the essential takeaways and bid farewell with some final thoughts.

Emphasizing the Importance of Consistent Breakfast Habits

Breakfast is often hailed as the most important meal of the day, and for good reason. It kickstarts your metabolism, replenishes your energy reserves, and sets the tone for the day ahead. With the scrumptious smoothie recipes presented in this eBook, you have a multitude of options to elevate your breakfast routine and ensure you start each day on a nourishing note.

Consistency is the key to reaping the full benefits of breakfast. Cultivate a habit of enjoying a wholesome smoothie in the morning, infusing your body with vitamins, minerals, and antioxidants. Whether you're a busy professional, a parent with little ones, or a health enthusiast, these recipes offer a quick and delicious solution to fuel your day.

Encouraging Readers to Explore and Enjoy Smoothie Recipes

Smoothies, as showcased in this eBook, are more than just beverages. They are canvases for culinary artistry, where you can experiment with flavors, colors, and textures. Embrace your creativity and make these recipes your own by tailoring them to your unique taste preferences and dietary requirements.

Beyond the recipes provided, there's a world of possibilities waiting to be discovered. Explore local fruits, seasonal produce, and superfoods specific to your region. Invite your family and friends to join in the smoothie-making adventure, fostering a sense of togetherness and wellness.

Final Thoughts and Closing Remarks

As we conclude this journey through "Healthy and Delicious Smoothie Recipes for Breakfast," let us part with gratitude for the abundance of nature's gifts. The ingredients we've incorporated into our smoothies offer a cornucopia of health benefits, each sip nurturing our bodies and minds.

Remember that healthy living is a continuous process, and our choices shape our well-being. By opting for nutritious breakfasts and incorporating smoothies into your daily routine, you've taken a positive step towards a healthier lifestyle.

May this eBook serve as a foundation for your culinary explorations and inspire you to embrace nourishing foods. As you embark on your smoothie adventures, let your imagination soar, and let your breakfast ritual be an expression of self-care and love.

Stay curious, stay playful, and stay well-fed with the delightful array of smoothies awaiting you. Cheers to a life filled with vibrant mornings and boundless energy!

With gratitude, prince emmanuel the author]

71

13

Cheers,

[Prince emmanuel]

Author of "Healthy and Delicious Smoothie Recipes for Breakfast"

thanks to all by readers hope this book will create a good impact in your life

please make sure your take a good breakfast

Thanks all!!!!!

ABOUT THE AUTHOR

prince emmanuel is a g

Healthy and Delicious Smoothie Recipes for Breakfast